David Oc

WHAT IS THE CAVEMAN DIET?

By

David Oc

©Copyright 2012 David Oc

ISBN-13: 978-1477495520

All rights reserved. No part of this publication may be reproduced or distributed in any form or by any means, electronic or mechanical, or stored in a database or retrieval system, without prior written permission from the publisher.

Disclaimer

This book is intended for informational use only. It is not meant to replace the advice of your healthcare provider. Before adopting any new diet or exercise program, consult with your healthcare provider. He or she can evaluate any new health regimen in light of your personal medical history.

David Oconner

Table of Contents

What is a Caveman Diet? (Paleo Diet)

Have you ever wondered why most pre-historic men and women are never depicted as fat and overweight slobs? Their depictions in mass media outlets such as movies, commercials endow them with Adonis-like proportions. So what is the ancient secret that lets Mr. Pre-historic He-Man keep his six-pack abs? Two words: Paleo diet.

What is a Paleo Diet?

How did this diet keep ancient man as healthy as an ox?

In regards to that question, paleo diet consisted mainly of fish, fruits and vegetables, and plenty of LEAN meat. This way of life ensured that these people had neither too much nor too little to eat. In other words, ancient man had the perfect recipe for being ripped.

However, with the discovery of fire, man began to cook foods that were once inedible. High-calorie items such as potatoes, beans and grains, which are toxic when raw, slowly became the staple in the ancient man's diet. These food items had several advantages: they can easily be stored for long periods of time, they are high in energy and calories, and their small size allowed them to be easily transported anywhere.

Advancing even further, man began to master the art of farming and agriculture. This enabled him to raise plants and animals easily to produce what was more than necessary for a balanced diet. A whole new one should first look at the lifestyle of the ancient ancestors. During their time, society was mainly composed of hunter-gatherers. These people had to hunt animals and gather plants for their food, which means they basically already expended a lot of energy just trying to eat. What's more, the range of food products emerged, from cow's milk to chicken eggs as a result.

Flash forward to modern times: there are now so many variety of foods cooked in an endless number of ways. The ingredients, instead of being natural, are being raised artificially and infused with man-made chemicals and preservatives. You can only guess the result: an alarmingly increasing rate of obesity spreading worldwide.

Now, why should you care what is a paleo diet all about? According to the proponents, man's genes are pre-programmed since ancient times to respond only to the foods found a paleo diet. Eating outside of these foods will eventually deteriorate the body of the individual. This explains why there are people who take vitamin supplements and try to de-toxify their systems- it's because they either had too much or too little of the essential nutrients their bodies needed.

With this in mind, it's no wonder that modern man's health is rapidly deteriorating. The paleo diet contains all that the body ever needs; everything else is unimportant. By knowing this fact, you can already try to regain a healthier you simply by changing your diet just like in the good old days.

Knowing what a paleo diet is and how it can greatly benefit your health, you can now try to modify your diet just like that of ancient man. With perseverance and hard work, your body can also become fit and lean, just as his was long ago.

Why a Caveman Paleolithic Diet Works in the Modern World

The modern mind can just imagine a day in the life of ancient man in pre-historic times. The world seemed so huge and hostile, and he had to be constantly on his tiptoes just survive each day. Threats from predators, fellow rivals, and the elements are regular occurrences in the life of ancient man.

Judging from all these things, ancient man needed a huge amount of energy to keep up. As he was known to be a hunter-gatherer in his time, his food needed to be plentiful, easy to gather, and easy to kill. However, they were not always plentiful and easy. Thus, ancient man consumed all he needed today to use as his energy to survive tomorrow. This cycle of energy consumption and expenditure sculpted ancient man's body like that of the gods: lean, chiselled, with barely an ounce of fat anywhere.

So what was the typical Paleo meal that ancient man subsisted on? First, there was certainly no amount of chemicals, preservatives, additives, etc. Sodium and sugar, for example, were a rarity in the ancient man's diet. Second, the food was not processed and refined as it is today; everything was cooked and prepared as it is. Lastly, ancient man's diet consisted of everything natural and healthy. As being fit and lean was a matter of life-and-death for them back then, they excluded everything else that their body didn't need.

What are the Foods That Make up a Typical Paleo Meal?

First, ancient man consumed a lot of meat. However, this is not the kind of meat found in supermarkets and delis today. The meat was derived from the wild game that they hunted. The meat was lean and natural and became the major staple in ancient man's diet. Aside from being lean, the meat also contained a good kind of fat: the omega-3 fatty acids, which are known to protect against heart diseases. Second to eating lean meat was the consumption of fish. Ancient man's diet consisted in a lot of fish; much more than today's modern diet.

Fish meat is also lean and provides an enormous amount of energy as well. Third, ancient man regularly consumed a lot of fruits and vegetables. These products grow in the wild and were regularly picked and gathered. In contrast to their farm-raised counterparts, they are chemical-free and contain a lot more essential nutrients. In particular, the wild vegetables contained a high amount of fiber, allowing ancient man to detoxify his systems quickly.

Also, wild fruits, being edible as well as rich in vitamins and antioxidants, were a favorite fare in the ancient man's diet. Lastly, nuts, being a great source of good fats also became a regular food item on the menu.

When man discovered fire for cooking, the caveman moved into a whole range of foods, many of which were unhealthy.

Increasing cases of obesity, heart diseases, diabetes, and other adverse health conditions continue to plague modern man due to his desire for an easier way of life.

People should return to a balanced lifestyle just like the one their ancestors had. This diet is available to anyone who wants to live a healthier way of life. Essentially, this is an exclusion diet, meaning you only eat what's acceptable and avoid those, which are not. However, if you stay long-term with this diet, then the benefits are enormous.

You can lose a great deal of weight do to the low-calories. This diet is generally free from allergens, meaning you can eat the food products as much as you want without incurring a hypersensitivity reaction. Also, your body will be able to de-toxify itself faster and become stronger against diseases as a result. Thanks to the diet, your immune system is far more resistant to diseases such as cancer, diabetes and other modern-day conditions.

Given the circumstances, people cannot hope to match the exact way of life that cavemen had in the past, including the diet. However, for the modern man, the caveman Paleolithic diet is definitely a very healthy, doable option.

Choosing Your Own Paleo Foods

Now that, you have decided to become fit and lean like the cavemen of the old days, you now have to decide your own Paleo foods. These foods will help you on your journey to fit and leaner body towards an overall healthier lifestyle. There are many kinds to food products to choose from, so you won't feel too restricted with this diet. What is important is that you stick to this diet long-term, and in return, you'll be rewarded with a healthier you.

However, before beginning, it is important to note that this is an exclusion diet, meaning all other foods, not on the list, cannot be eaten. Fast foods, processed and refined foods, carbonated drinks, etc. are forbidden. These food products contain more calories you'll need, while having little nutritional value. They will short-change your body, leaving you more prone to obesity, diseases, and poor mental health.

First on the Paleo foods list is the meat. You can consume as much meat as you want for the three meals of the day; however, the meat should be lean. For the preparation, the meat can be cooked through broiling, roasting, baking, or sautéing. Never, ever cook the meat in the deep fryer as it will result in too much fat and oil content being mixed with the meat. Examples of good, lean meat include wild deer, turkey, boar, and game fowls. However, for those who live in an urban setting, then you should choose the freshest meat you can find at the deli or supermarket. Examples include skinless chicken breasts, trimmed lean pork, and organ meats such as livers, tongues, and marrows. Duck and goose eggs can also be consumed as a source of lean protein.

For the fish and seafood, any commercially available species will do. Examples include tuna, trout, mackerel and salmon. Good seafood includes crabs, shrimps, lobster, and shellfish. However, remember to avoid those products that have already been processed such as those sardines and anchovies you find in cans. Also, make sure that they have either been caught at sea, or grown naturally without the use of artificial feeds, which may contain chemicals and other harmful substances. Lastly, avoid these products if you are allergic to any of them. There are plenty of other alternative healthy food products to choose from.

Then there are fruit and vegetables. These food products have a high amount of essential nutrients and help the body detoxify itself faster thanks to the high amount of fiber content. Fruits of any kind can be consumed, while green, leafy vegetables are very ideal for a healthy body. Also, nuts such as almonds and pecans have a high amount of good fats called Omega-6 fats and should be included. However, not all fruits and vegetables are beneficial.

Remember to avoid fruits that have been dried and canned because they may contain high amounts of glucose, and vegetables such as potatoes and yams, because they have high caloric content and little nutritional value. Also, it's best to avoid nuts if you are allergic to them.

With so many Paleo foods to choose from, you'd be hard-pressed not to remain with this diet. After all, it's you who can benefit the most if you stick to the program.

The Paleo Diet Eating Plan

The Paleo-diet-eating-plan solution is what you need if your goal is to achieve and maintain a healthier body. The concept is simple and straightforward. Your approach to diet should be one like the cave men where you eat only natural and organic food and avoid processed food.

Following this plan, you should not eat grains, dairy, and their products, as they are not suitable for the body's food consumption. It was only during the agricultural and industrial revolutions that human dietary habits drastically changed to accommodate these produce and products.

The result of these drastic changes in the eating habits of human is not favorable to the health. In fact, according to the Paleo diet program, these dietary changes have damaging effects such as exposing the body to deadly diseases and serious health problems resulting to a shortened lifespan.

The Paleo Basics

Under the Paleo program, you will eat food designed for human consumption before all these revolutions changed the dietary habit. You will have to avoid all processed food. The Paleo diet believes that processing contaminates food with chemicals and toxic substances that are harmful and damaging to the body.

Instead, the diet promotes that eating of natural and organic food, especially fruits and vegetables that you can eat at their most natural condition even in unlimited proportions. This way, your body is free from contaminants, preservatives, and toxins from processed food.

How to Make the Diet Work

You can follow this simple Paleo-diet-eating-plan solution to start benefitting from the program:

- Create your Paleo meal plans. Remember to keep it simple and easy to follow to ensure greater success. The key to success is in planning your Paleo meals.

- Make sure that all of the necessary ingredients are available. This will sustain your momentum in following your meals.

- Begin your diet by preparing the food that you like and are familiar with. As soon as you get accustomed to your Paleo diet plan, you can then start to experiment and introduce new food gradually but steadily.

- Enjoy eating your Paleo meals. Visualize how healthy your body can be and how you can live longer by sticking to your Paleo diet regimen.

Tips to Increase Success

- Use the Paleo Food Lists so you will have an easy reference on what food to eat and what food to avoid;

- Your Paleo meals should begin with the easiest recipes of dishes that you like the eat the most;

- Read Paleo books that will show in easy systematic manner how you can get the most from this diet.

Benefits From Paleo Meals

By following the Paleo diet, you will be able to train yourself from avoiding processed food and reducing the amount of toxins that enter your body as a result. Since you are re-learning to eat only natural and organic food, you enjoy a healthier diet that can reduce your excess weight, make you feel better, and make you look good.

More importantly, if you want to stay away from degenerative diseases including the deadly cancer, then you must start your Paleo-diet-eating-plan right now.

Paleo meals bring many health benefits to the body. If you are attracted to processed food because they are quick and easy to prepare, you will certainly be delighted to know that meals under the Paleo diet can be as quick and easy as processed and instant meals. There is no reason not to benefit from the Paleo diet program.

How to Prepare the Meals

The meals under the Paleo program require simple preparation. Most of the meals are quick to prepare. Complete Paleo meals usually need only twenty (20) minutes or less to prepare. The methods are easy- you boil, bake, stew, poach or fry. You just have to use the food or ingredients that are in the Paleo food lists.

There is no limit to what you can do with this meal as long as you follow what is in the list. You can experiment and come up with your own gourmet dishes that will satisfy your gastronomic taste. Preparation does not have to be complicated, you can always prepare quick but savoury meals playing with the Paleo food lists and referencing some Paleo books.

Useful Tips and Techniques

Here, are some useful tips and techniques to get the most out of your Paleo meals:

Clear your kitchen and your home from all processed, junk, and instant food. This will prevent you from temptations and help you to focus more on following your healthy diet.

Imagine yourself being transported back to the ancient times when humankind's Palaeolithic ancestors lived. Would you not want to have their strong bodies and live longer as they did? Use this as your motivation.

Map out your meals. You have the option to create a daily meal plan or a weekly meal plan depending on what is most convenient to you. Make sure that the ingredients are handy and readily available when you need them for preparation.

Savour your meals. Make your healthy eating a habit.

Health Benefits

As soon as you are able to develop the Paleo program as your habit, you will appreciate the many health benefits your meals bring to your body. Your meals will activate and strengthen your body's natural defence and protection against diseases, and you will feel how your body becomes stronger and more energized.

Here, are just some of the health benefits you can gain from your Paleo diet meals:

Have an enhanced immune system that shields your body from diseases and other damages caused by free radicals and harmful bacteria.

Increase in energy. You will feel stronger, and more energized, to do the things that you want and need to do.

Lose unnecessary weight. The meals will help you lose your excess weight and from there keep and maintain your recommended or ideal weight.

Enjoy clear skin. Beauty begins with clear skin, and with these meals at work, you will not only feel good, but you will even look better, with clearer and healthier skin.

Plan your Paleo meals right now and see how you will be able to maximize the benefits you can gain from your new diet program.

The Paleo Food Lists

Discover the Paleo food lists that will empower you to stay healthy and live longer. The lists are part of the Paleo diet. This diet program is heavily inspired by the Palaeolithic age where you eat natural food and avoid processed food.

The lists contain the food that you can eat under the program. If you look at the lists, you will note how you can eat practically all food as long as they are natural and save for some food high in carbohydrates such as grains, dairies and their derivatives.

Food You Can Eat

Under the Paleo diet program, the recommended food to eat consists of lean meat, eggs, fruits and vegetables. The meat can come from beef, pork, lamb, goat, horse, chicken, turkey, duck, as well as from fish and more provided they are lean and healthy meat.

When it comes to fruits and vegetables, you are encouraged to eat all fruits. As for vegetables, you should only limit your consumption of vegetables rich in starch such as potatoes. Starchy vegetables are high in carbohydrates. The body stores and converts unused carbohydrates as fats.

Food You Should Eat in Moderation

There are certain food groups in the Paleo food lists that you should consume in moderation. These include oils (although you should prefer oils from olive and canola) where you are allowed up to 4 tablespoons of consumption in a day.

You may drink caffeinated beverages such as coffee, tea, and soda drinks in scant amount. If you are to drink beer, wine and spirits, you should be frugal in drinking and only up to one bottle of beer, or two small glasses of wine, or 4 ounces of spirits.

Food You Should Avoid

The Paleo diet does not allow the consumption of dairies like milk, butter, cheese, ice cream, and yoghurt. You must not also consume any form of grains like wheat, rye, oats, barley, or corn, as well as any type of beans like soybeans.

Any food that requires processing or contains preservative and chemicals is strictly prohibited and has no place under this diet program. The way to go to is to consume organic and natural food.

This is because processing of food is seen by the Paleo diet as highly dangerous to one's health that lead you to life threatening diseases such as the deadly 'C'. This is with strong basis from several reputable studies that have established the link between consumption of processed food and the occurrence of cancers.

While most are quick to blame the saturated fats, found in processed food, two other culprits make processed food unhealthy and dangerous. One is toxic substances and the other is the contaminants present in processed food.

Have you not wondered why people from the olden times, during the Palaeolithic age, have lived a hundred years despite the absence of medical breakthroughs? The answer is in the food they eat. By following the Paleo food lists, you now have unravelled the secret to good health and long life.

Paleo Diet Athletes – How to Get the Athletic Body You Desire

Paleo Diet Athletes is a diet program that anyone who wishes to have a body like that of an athlete can easily follow. While the diet program primarily caters to athletes, you can also choose to use it to improve your body built and enjoy an athletic body you have longed desired.

Gaining Muscles

One of the envied features of athletes is their strong muscles. The Paleo diet for athletes can help you build and maintain robust muscles, and here is how you can achieve it:

- You need to work out your muscles. If you want your muscles to grow, you need to train them to stimulate their growth. You can do this at home with appropriate exercises intended to build and strengthen the muscles. You can also choose to enrol in a muscle- building program.

- Following the Paleo diet, eat adequate amount of lean meat. This will supply your muscles the protein it needs to grow stronger. Your Paleo meals should therefore focus on eating more of high quality lean meat to increase the supply of protein the muscles need.

- Apart from protein, your body also need calories, which you can get from fish or fish oil supplements. Fish oil contains anti-inflammatory elements that will prevent you to experience joint pains. It will also speed up relaxation of your muscles after your training.

- You must have your Paleo snack meals ready. Your Paleo snacks will satisfy your hunger in between your main meals. It will also provide your body with the additional calories it needs to build strong muscles.

- Paleo Diet Athletes also encourages you to get enough rest and relaxation you can gain from sleeping. It is during sleep that your body recovers and recharges to get ready for the next day's training. This is also an environment needed by the body to grow your muscles at its optimum.

Advantages

The Paleo diet for athletes has several advantages. By supplying the body with nutrients to strengthen the muscles and physique, any athlete or wannabe can max out his performance. The diet ensures that the body has the necessary supply of protein the muscles need to grow and sustain its strength.

Eating the Paleo meals also restores the ideal acid-alkaline ratio in the body. Excessive acids in the body damages muscle tissues. The alkaline found in Paleo meals neutralizes excess acids and restores the normal balance to prevent damages to the muscle tissues.

Another important advantage is that athletes and wannabes can become more resistant to ailments and diseases as the Paleo diet meals strengthen the immune system. Getting sick is the last thing in an athlete's mind, and when the immune system is working at its best, there's no way that ailments or diseases can win.

What is best about the Paleo Diet Athletes is that you can customize it to fit your needs. As an athlete requiring special nutritional needs, there are instances where you need to consume carbohydrates and starch. While Paleo diet promotes the avoidance of carbohydrates and starch, it can allow its consumption in times that best fits the athletic training requirements to build strong muscles and get the athletic body you desire.

How Paleo Books Can Make the Paleo Diet More Exciting

Paleo books can transform your Paleo diet into a gastronomic delight. The books will also reveal the natural secrets to healthy living and longer life from the Palaeolithic age where people lived beyond one hundred years. There are several authors and books showing the relevance of going back to the basics in the consumption of food.

A Look at the Paleo Diet

The Paleo diet, also known as the caveman diet, is a program that pushes the return to basic eating habits such as that of the Paleo people or the cave men. Remember that during those times, people eat natural and organic food for lack of technology to process food. These people get to live an average of one hundred years old despite the absence of medical technology.

Logically, in order to improve one's health and increase the lifespan, you would go back to those ancient days and how ancestors survive through their diet. This is the principle behind the Paleo diet expounded on several books written about it. You eat natural and organic food and avoid processed food; you stay healthy and live longer.

The Food to Eat

If you think the food to eat under the Paleo diet advocacy is bland and tasteless as they are natural and organic, you have to rethink. While you can easily label healthy diet programs as boring and dull, the Paleo diet may just turn out to be a culinary pleasure. There are several things you can do with Paleo foods to satisfy your taste, without having to subject your food to processing.

There are Paleo books that will show you the complete Paleo food lists and various gourmet recipes you can prepare. With these recipes, you can easily transform a typical diet into one that is magical to your taste while enabling you to stay healthy and fit. The Paleo diet can combine your taste for good food and the need to stay fit, trim, and healthy.

The Health Benefits

You will also know from the books how the Paleo diet can bring you multiple health benefits. You will understand how the diet works to prevent progressive ailments such as cardiovascular diseases, hypertension, and joint pains among others and how these diseases relate to the damage done by processed food on your digestive system.

Several studies reveal that cave men rarely suffered, or none at all, from degenerative health problems. Back then, these men did not suffer from bone loss or inflammation and were healthy and strong despite their primitive environment. There are also studies conducted and clinical testing made on modern-day individuals who were placed in similar primitive conditions and environments, especially with their food consumption, and were found to produce favorable results of good health.

All these things, including how you can achieve an athletic body structure though healthy diet, you will find from the Paleo book, "Paleo Solution Diets" at Lifestyles100 web site.

Get yours today and start to enjoy living a healthy life where you can look forward to a longer life.

About the Author

David Oc has been writing and publishing books on many of his varied interests. He has books on topics such as Power Juicing, The Paleo Diet, Sugar Gliders, Iguanas, Cichlid fish, Fitness, Lactose Intolerance, waterproofing a basement, probiotics, dog and cat training, Minecraft and more.

www.ingramcontent.com/pod-product-compliance
Lightning Source LLC
Chambersburg PA
CBHW070123010626
45794CB00012B/1256